The body is a temple —
You taught me how to
take good care of it.
I am forever grateful.
Dana

God, Where Are You When I Need You?
An Atheist's Search for Faith and Healing

Dana Watts

Disclaimer

I have tried to recreate events and conversations from my memories of them. In order to protect their privacy, I have changed the names of individuals and some of their identifying characteristics.

Copyright © 2015 by Dana Watts

All Rights Reserved

Cover photo by Dana Watts.
Photo taken on St. James Way, Najera, Spain - 2015.
Cover design by Angelee Nuti

Published by Amazon Publishing

No part of this publication may be reproduced, stored in a retrieval system, or transmitted in any form by any means, electronic, mechanical, photocopy, recording or otherwise, without the prior written permission of the publisher, except for brief quotations in critical reviews or articles.

To Laura and Diana

You encouraged me every step of the way.

*And now abide faith, hope, love, these three;
but the greatest of these is love.*
1 Corinthians 13:13

Table of Contents

News 7

Father John 15

You Have Cancer 25

Surgery 31

Surgery - Part 2 39

Rabbi Moishe 43

Service for Healing 53

Pastor Smith 61

Father Maximilian 69

Rabbi Cassel 79

The Ghost in the Machine 89

Fear and Trembling 95

Father Maximilian - Reprise 99

Nathan 107

The Dream 117

Faith 123

Notes 131

Personal Thoughts 133

News

When the bottom drops out of your life, you are never the same again. You may get up and dust yourself off, you may limp away, you may walk away, but things are irrevocably changed.

⁓

April, 2014. A lump in my left breast. I think I am imagining things. There is so much lumpiness in the breast, it's like weird cottage cheese. How can you tell anything? I am sure it's nothing! But I don't think it was there a few days ago ... I am not sure. It's sore. Is it supposed to hurt? Now I am scared! What the heck is it? Was it there yesterday? I am sure it's nothing. There is no family history of cancer. We just don't have a cancer gene. What a relief! I scared myself for a moment. I will call the doctor in the morning. I know she will be reassuring: "Of course you are fine! Such a silly worry. There is no family history of cancer. You have a healthy lifestyle: you are a vegetarian - everyone should eat like you! You don't smoke, you exercise, you do yoga. You are the poster child for a lifestyle that protects you from cancer." Ok, I feel better. I will be able to sleep tonight. Tomorrow I will call the doctor.

⌒

"I'm not going to lie to you. We need to do a biopsy. It looks very concerning." *What does that mean? I don't understand. Why does she think I need a biopsy? I am protected by good genes. I am scared and I cry. I have done everything the right way. Just the other day in the paper there was an article about breast health with a checklist of things to do to protect you from breast cancer. I do them all! A+. I am sure she's mistaken.* I cry again. It hurts and I feel afraid.

⌒

June 2nd. "I am sorry to have to tell you, the biopsy came back positive. You have breast cancer."
The bottom fell out of my world. Everything I knew disappeared in an instant. All the things that made sense in my life became incomprehensible. Everything felt despairingly pointless.

The next few months were the darkest in my life. How could I go on when nothing made sense? How comforting the routines and habits of my life had been and how empty and cold it all turned when they were stripped away with one stroke!

Why? Why did this happen? I am sobbing yet again because my heart is broken, because my soul hurts. *I don't understand! I need to understand. Why? Why me?* But there is no answer. I will never have an answer. I want things to make sense. But nothing makes sense, and my predictable life feels completely out of control. If all the things I did have not protected me, then how do I move forward? If what I did did not matter, what matters then?

I felt disoriented and lost; I felt ashamed. As a psychologist I took great pride in having my life together, being in control, having all the answers. Yet there I was, reeling and unable to cope. I felt that I lost all my credibility. How could I counsel others about how to manage themselves when I couldn't manage my own self?

Before cancer, I was in control. I knew what I wanted and pursued it with passion and determination, whatever it was. Self-control and life control, I had it all. But three little words, "you have cancer," changed all that, and I was in free fall. The control that I cherished so deeply was an illusion. Cancer put things in perspective: we cannot control life as we might control a mechanical toy. And just like that, with the illusion of control stripped away, I had nothing but fear and emptiness and darkness. And, for the first time, my spirit yearned for something greater than me, than this life.

I listened to people in the support groups who shared their stories of pain and illness, yet spoke with such lightness and courage and hope. They talked about their faith and about God and the strength that He gave them. They were filled with serenity and peace. How could that be? Their stories of cancer terrified me. Were they not scared? How could they be so calm? It made no sense to me, but it filled me with wonder and yearning and an unquenchable desire to feel like them. How wonderful it must be to believe that God is at your side, that you are not alone, no matter how scared you feel and what challenges you face.

⁓

I grew up in communist Romania during the repressive dictatorship of Ceausescu. Churches were closed and torn down. To be religious or, even worse, to go to church, was a dangerous thing. Hymns were sung to the dictator not to God. There was no God. You did not need God when you had the Great Leader. And, if that were not sufficient to make one's heart dead to belief, both my parents were atheists. I grew up deriding religious beliefs as foolish and simple. What was the point of religion and faith? If you believe in yourself and work hard, you can make anything happen. You don't need a higher power!

Until you do.

I was raised to scoff at those who had faith and believed, yet part of me always looked at them with envy. How nice it must be to feel that comfort, to have a personal God who cares and takes an interest in you! I yearned for that comfort and faith. I felt like the child who looks in but is not invited to the party. Everyone is joyful and happy, while I remain outside, never to be asked in.

I look back and see myself as a young child, perhaps 5 or 6 years old. I remember going inside and telling my parents that I wanted to be baptized. A well-meaning neighbor had told me that all children should be baptized and that when they are, they get to have a godmother who helps them believe in God and buys them a present every year on their birthday. The things she said seemed to me as beautiful and magical as a fairytale. Decades later I can still see the scene: a little girl determinedly announcing her decision to be baptized and just as swiftly being shut down and threatened with corporal punishment if she ever brought up such a thing again. I remember being crushed by that denial, feeling as though the magic was forever erased from my life. Looking at that event with adult eyes, it feels seminal in its impact: though you no longer think of it consciously, it leaves an indelible mark of disappointment that haunts you for the rest of your life: you are not like the other children who are baptized, there is no magic, you have no God. To be an atheist is to be eternally alone.

Father John

My journey of spiritual discovery started with Father John, the Catholic priest at my friend Ellen's church. She felt that he could help me.

Being atheist, I have had no church affiliation. I have been to church a few times in my life, mostly out of curiosity, sometimes out of obligation. Interestingly, I remember each experience quite clearly. I remember the liturgy at the Romanian Orthodox church in Romanian and in English. I remember the incense and the chants and the vestments. But I mostly remember a certain exhilaration, which was strange and unexplainable.

I remembered my last trip to Romania, though I hadn't thought of it in years. I remembered traveling to a monastery in the mountains where the relics of a saint, who had only recently died, were buried. I was sick that day with severe nausea from the hours of driving up and down winding, mountainous roads. "Drink some holy water," my cousin urged me, "it will settle your stomach right up." I did.

I drank some holy water, and felt better minutes later. "I told you it would help," my cousin declared triumphantly. "Yes, you did and you were right," I responded agreeably, but in my mind, I knew better. I was sure it was the effect of the mountain spring water and the solid ground under my feet. Yet, in spite of myself, I felt a kind of eerie magic, a strange sense of otherworldly holiness all around me.

I remember the Baptist sermons of Mr. Kinsey who sponsored my family's entry into this country. At first they felt tedious and tiresome, but my spotty English mastery probably accounted for much of it because, as time passed, I started to find them soothing. I found myself sometimes thinking of the homily of the previous Sunday. There was comfort and inspiration in what Mr. Kinsey said.

I remember, too, the sabbath service with our friends in Connecticut and the beautiful voice of the cantor. I remember thinking "from his mouth to God's ear." What a strange thought for an atheist!

And I remember a smattering of wedding, baptism, and funeral services. For believers, everything from birth to death is filled with community and comforting rituals. What is there to embrace the atheist? What can the atheist embrace? Emptiness and loneliness do not give much comfort.

When life was good, before cancer, I gave little thought to God. I had little time or need for Him. All was well, I had everything under control and life was full to the brim with activities and commitments. Occasionally, though, a desire for something bigger, a feeling of yearning would break through, especially when witnessing others coping with loss. Their faith that God was there for them, that he would give them the strength to bear the burden felt mystifying to me, but awe inspiring as well. Then I wished for such calmness and strength of spirit. Then I would think, "how wonderful it must be to have that kind of belief, how comforting and reassuring." But then life with its incessant demands would return, clamoring for my attention, and those thoughts would be quickly forgotten or pushed away. Until cancer happened and life stopped.

How does one cope with cancer, a thing so fearsome that people refer to it as "the big C," as if the word itself could bring on the disease or cast an evil spell? The mere sound makes one's blood run cold and fills the brave with terror! It strikes a chord of fear that seems as primal and instinctive as the fear of snakes. Yet survival rates have increased dramatically over the past 20 years. Breast cancer, especially, has become a success story. A breast cancer diagnosis was a death sentence in the early 1900s, now even for stage 3 diagnoses the survival rate is 73%. I knew all this and I took comfort in it. And I knew that I was in great hands, all the doctors and nurses expertly and efficiently handling every facet of my treatment. But who was there to care for my broken heart, my suffering spirit? No amount of chemotherapy or radiation could restore my sense of trust, my faith in life. And as I struggled with the unanswerable, I realized that perhaps I could find spiritual healing by talking to people whose job it is to cure the spirit.

⁓

I called Father John, with some trepidation, but with hope as well. Would he talk to me? Was there anything that he could say to help my tormented spirit? Would he condemn me when he learned that I did not believe in God? I did not know what to expect and I
felt nervous.

We agreed to meet on a Saturday morning. It was a dark and gloomy day in November. A thin, chilly rain was falling, mirroring my somber mood. On the 40 minute drive to meet with him, I had time to think of an introduction. What should I say? What did I want? I want to have faith. I want to believe. I want there to be light in the darkness. Is there hope for me? Is it too late? I am reminded of the terrible experiments with kittens in which their eyes were sewn shut to find out what happens to their vision. After a few weeks, the sutures were removed and their eyes opened, but they could not see. They were functionally blind. Though their eyes and brain were perfectly healthy, they could not see. Because they were not allowed to see when their brain was forming connections, they missed the window for developing sight. Am I like those kittens? Is the window for developing a spiritual self closed to me forever? Is that why I cannot understand what faith is? Because my spiritual eyes were sewn shut when I was a child?

"There is no deadline on faith," said Father John simply. "There is no time limit or age limit. Faith can come at any age. All you need is a readiness and, clearly, you have that readiness, or else you wouldn't be here talking to me."

"What do I have to do to get faith?" I asked

"Faith is not a thing that you get. It is not the end result of a formula. There is no recipe or particular thing you have to do. It is not a task you have to accomplish. It's not something you control. All you need is an openness, a willingness to be touched by God. A willingness to ask God to enter your life. I think in some ways you have been ready for it for a long time. You told me you used to read a picture Bible to your children. Why else would you have read it? I know, you wanted them to know the stories of the Bible, but you could have taught them the same stories in other ways. You have been ready for a long time, you just did not know it."

"I hear everything you are saying and I understand your words, but at the very same time, I don't understand at all what this means. I want to, but I can't."

I continued: "I used to read a book to my children, I think it was a bible story too, about the farmer who was sowing seeds. But the seeds were falling on hard, crusted ground. Those seeds could not sprout, so they died. I feel like that dry, crusted ground. The seeds that you sow cannot break through. Your words cannot penetrate. I feel like the parched, hard ground."

"The wonderful thing about faith", said Father John quietly, "is that you do not have to struggle so. All you have to do is allow it to enter your life. And for that all you need is quietness, a time and place where you can pray for that readiness and openness, and God will hear you."

"How does one pray the right way? Is praying like meditation?"

"There is no right way or wrong way to pray," he replied. "There is no formula for that either. Praying is speaking to God, and knowing, having the faith that God is listening to you. Praying is asking God to help you with your readiness so that faith may grow within. Praying is being quiet and allowing the Spirit to enter your soul. You cannot force it or rush it. All you can do is be open.

"In our culture we expect results, but faith is not

about results. Faith is quiet acceptance and peace. Pray every day, find a quiet place and time and ask God for guidance. Read the Bible; just read in it, see what resonates for you, what attracts you. Ask yourself what meaning it has for you, why you were attracted to that particular reading and allow faith to take root and grow within you. We can meet again if you wish to continue." And with that we parted.

I did dig out the Bible when I returned home. I wanted to be a good student and start on the journey of openness. As Father John suggested, I opened the Bible at random to read a passage, but the passage I opened to seemed far from random:

> *"The Lord is my shepherd; I shall not want.*
> *He makes me to lie down in green pastures;*
> *He leads me beside the still waters.*
> *He restores my soul;*
> *He leads me in the paths of righteousness*
> *For His name's sake.*
> *Yea, though I walk through the valley*
> *of the shadow of death,*
> *I will fear no evil, for you are with me;*
> *Your rod and Your staff, they comfort me.*
> *You prepare a table before me in the*
> *presence of my enemies;*

> *You anoint my head with oil;*
> *My cup runs over.*
> *Surely goodness and mercy will follow me*
> *All the days of my life;*
> *And I will dwell in the house of the Lord*
> > *to the end of my days."*
>
> > Psalm 23:1-6

Was this a message? It certainly was a refreshing drink of water to a parched soul. Coincidence or message? Father John urged me to be open, so I allowed myself to imagine that it was a message.

Father John had suggested that I read the Bible to see what "speaks" to me. He seemed certain that the Bible would help me discover the fountain of faith within me and that gave me hope. But as I pondered his words, a different thought came to me. Could the Bible help me with something else, equally, if not even more, pressing: coming to terms with the scourge that is cancer? I wanted to be able to "lie down in green pastures" again, to rest "beside the still waters." Cancer had robbed me of those things that were happy and soothing. Since the diagnosis, no gentleness inhabited my spirit; every step I took was "through the valley of the shadow of death." Could God speak to me through the Bible and help "restore my soul?" I embarked on this quest with an urgency that might have made Father John frown. After all, he warned me that "faith was not about doing." But, for the first time in many months, I felt an excitement that I had thought was lost to me. Father John had given me a key, a key that could open the door to freedom and peace.

> *"If anyone is in Christ, he is a new creation:*
> *old things have passed away;*
> *behold, all things have become new."*
>
> *2 Corinthians 5:17*

You Have Cancer

"You have cancer," three words that caused darkness and despair to descend in an instant, like a heavy curtain in the middle of a play. No curtain calls, no rousing ovations, no thunderous claps followed; only stunned astonishment. "It must be a mistake!" was the only thought I could muster. One hears occasinally of test results being accidentally switched, lab work specimens mistakenly labeled. I clung desperately to that thought, yet I knew that I could not think away the tumor that was clearly there in my left breast. The days that followed, I moved around in a daze, unable to wrap my head around those words: "you have cancer."

The mornings and the nights were the hardest. In those first few days, by morning time I would forget. I'd wake up ready to face the day with the excitement I always had, but that lasted mere moments. The thought quickly returned, "you have cancer!" more terrifying each time because with every passing day, the fear and the darkness grew stronger. And the nights, well the nights were filled with their own special kind of frightening darkness. It was then that all the fears and the questions rushed in like an avalanche: *Will I die? Will the treatment work? Will I be very sick? Has it spread? What will happen to me? Will I see my children established in life? Are my days numbered? Why did this happen to me? What have I done to deserve this?* When everything you know is suddenly turned upside down, what are you left with but questions and doubts and emptiness? Cancer interrupted my life. No, it brought my life to a complete halt.

The statistics on breast cancer show that 1 in 8 women will be diagnosed with breast cancer in their lifetime and that the two highest risk factors are being a woman and being older than 50. I have both risk factors, but even so, I landed in the minority group of women who got cancer. Why me? Why us, the 1 in 8? We are a mixture of nature and nurture. For me nature was not an issue - no one in my family tree had been ever afflicted by cancer. So it must be nurture - something about my life put me in that group. Yes, all kinds of environmental factors increase the risk: chemicals, pesticides, toxins. But we are all exposed to them. In fact, I was exposed less as a vegetarian who was conscientious about living a clean and healthy lifestyle. How could I make sense of this thing that happened to me? I felt so overwhelmed. I was standing, small and insignificant, at the foot of a mountain that felt insurmountable, that blocked all future paths of my life.

> *"Because of your unbelief, for assuredly,*
> *I say to you, if you have faith as a mustard*
> *seed, you will say to this mountain,*
> *'Move from here to there,' and it will move;*
> *and nothing shall be impossible for you."*
> *Matthew 17:20*

The days were busy after the diagnosis. With one short statement, "You have cancer," my life stopped being my own. I cleared my schedule of everything that earlier had felt essential. The countless doctor's appointments and tests now took priority. The usual places that I frequented were replaced by doctors' offices and hospitals and labs and waiting rooms

I had a favorite seat in the waiting room of the oncology department: right in front of reception, where I could hear the cheerful voices of the receptionists and their warm greeting to every patient that checked in. Before I became a "regular," I was afraid of that waiting room. I thought that people would be sad and grim and somber, and that the receptionists would speak in hushed voices, as though at a wake. But their cheerfulness gave me hope, that they did no write us off, that there was life on the other side of this terrible ordeal.

―

The surgeon recommended a lumpectomy. I was relieved because I did not want to face a mastectomy. She said other things, too: that one in four women require a second surgery or even a mastectomy to remove additional tissue, if a clean margin was not achieved on the first try. I didn't concern myself much with it. After all, seventy five percent was pretty good odds. A lumpectomy felt like a reasonable compromise. I had cancer, but after the surgery and treatment, my body would be intact, as if nothing ever happened. I would have my life back.

Surgery

When the day of surgery finally came, it was relief that I mainly felt. The tumor felt like an alien that had taken control of my body and my life. The lumpectomy would remove it, and, if the cancer hadn't spread to the lymph nodes, I would be done and this terrible chapter in my life would be over.

I had had surgeries before, so the process felt familiar: IV's, waiting in the pre-op room, nurses and doctors stopping by to discuss the procedure, to take vitals, to ask questions, to reassure me. I meditated and focused on my breath while I waited, and visualized an easy surgery and fast healing. When the anesthesiologist came, I was ready, and then I went out like a light.

"The doctor said she felt really good about the surgery," my daughter told me as soon as I came out of anesthesia. "You had two positive lymph nodes, and she removed a total of eight, but she said that it went well." What a relief! It was the good news I had hoped for after all the weeks of fear and worry.

A week of recovery, some pain that was surprisingly tolerable without medication, some mild unpleasantness with the drain tube, but all in all I felt upbeat. I looked forward to meeting with the oncologist to find out what the plan of action would be. "Let's get the job done," has always been my motto.

⁓

"Could you come in earlier in the day to have the drain removed?," asked the nurse on the phone.

"Happily! I am ready to be rid of this ball and chain!"

I was nervous waiting for the nurse. I had heard that pulling out the drain hurts like the dickens, so I sat in the air-conditioned room feeling hot in spite of the cold air. *How bad could it be, after all? Besides, it will only last a second. Surely I can handle it!*

I was surprised to see the surgeon come in. I did not have an appointment with her. And then my heart stopped. I saw it in her eyes, as clearly as I could see the poster of a tranquil beach scene behind her: she had
bad news.

"Dana, I have some bad news. The tumor I removed did not have clean margins. We have to do another surgery." She said more things, but I could only hear her in patches: "another lumpectomy," "would be disfiguring," "mastectomy," "reconstruction." "If it were me, that is what I would choose."

The proverbial rug was once again pulled out from under me, and there I was— overwhelmed and scared and angry. Yet again I could not wrap my mind around the news. This cannot be! The odds were in my favor! I was filled with rage and disbelief. She made a mistake! Why didn't she do it right the first time? She said everything went well, she felt positive that she got it all! I was so angry with her; I needed someone to blame, an outlet for my rage. I could not face another surgery! The tenuous balance I had reached after the lumpectomy crumbled like a house of cards in a puff of wind.

More days of crying and fear and questions. *Why is this happening to me? I have been a good person! I don't understand anything. Is it my fault? Do I deserve this? Will I die? I can't deal with this anymore.*
I don't feel strong enough to handle yet another surgery.

Three weeks to wait for the surgery— an eternity, while my imagination ran amok. Every twitch in my body made me think that the cancer was spreading. Pain behind my knees made me imagine that the cancer had already metastasized to lymph nodes there. I tried to do deep breathing exercises and visualize how with each breath the cancer cells were swept away, their DNA disintegrating, blown apart by the breath of relaxation that packed the punch of a typhoon. Occasionally I found a place of mental quiet, but most times I failed miserably. I had no understanding and I could find no peace. I was a bit of flotsam caught in a sea of feelings, tossed around by the powerful waves of emotions and questions. Why? Why? Why? There was no answer and no peace. I felt alone.

> *"Blessed is a man who finds wisdom*
> *And the man who sees discernment;*
> *For the profits gained from wisdom are better*
> *Than the treasures of gold and silver.*
> *And wisdom is more valuable than*
> *precious stones."*
>
> *Proverbs 3:13-14*

I read the Bible and meditated on what I read. Some days I opened it to a random page and read where my eyes fell. Other days I took suggestions from an old calendar I had with Bible quotes for each day and read the whole section suggested.

How will I know when I have faith? How does it feel to have faith? Is it a feeling of deep relaxation? Is it happiness? Is it peacefulness? I have no frame of reference to judge and know.

I felt like I was waiting in a station for someone to arrive, not knowing whom I was meeting, only that he would appear at my side, and I would know it when I saw him. *But how would I know? In the endless stream of feelings running through my mind, which one is faith? Will I recognize it when it arrives? I do not know,* so I turn to the Bible for an answer. By accident (or was there design in this as well?), I stumbled on the parable of the farmer sowing seeds, the very story I had read to my children so many years ago:

> *"Now he who received seed among the thorns is he who hears the word, but the cares of this world and the deceitfulness of riches choke the word and he becomes unfruitful. But he who received seed on the good ground is he who hears the word, and understands it; who indeed bears fruit and produces, some a hundredfold, some sixty, some thirty."*
>
> *Matthew 13:22-23*

I took the message to mean that I must persist. Though my heart was filled with doubt, perhaps one day, faith would grow there instead, and the weeds of doubt would wither away.

> *"The Lord stood with me and strengthened me so that the message might be preached fully through me...And the Lord will deliver me from every evil work and preserve me for His heavenly kingdom."*
>
> *2 Timothy 4:17-18*

Surgery – Part 2

How strange is the experience of time! On vacation, three weeks fly by in the blink of an eye, but three weeks of living with cancer and waiting for the mastectomy move with the speed of a glacier. Fear was a daily companion, but I was grateful that life's demands were forcing me to look outward rather than dwell on possibilities. Things had to be done, a wedding to be planned. My daughter was getting married three days before my surgery. Not a minute could be wasted on idle thoughts and preoccupations. It was good to be busy planning and thinking about something that was beautiful and life-affirming. The last minute preparations, the food, the flowers, the seating, the arranging, everything needed attention. Little time was left for thoughts of cancer, but fear, like a dark and silent shadow, was always at my side.

The wedding was beautiful - a celebration of love and life and hope. Good friends and family, food and music, dancing and cheer, and a gloriously sunny day! That day, for those few hours, cancer did not have a place at the table. Happiness and joy were king!

> *"And God is able to make all grace abound toward you, that you, always having all sufficiency in all things, may abound for every good work."*
>
> *2 Corinthians 9:8*

With the wedding over, there was nothing to focus on but the upcoming surgery. *A mastectomy! How will it feel to have only one breast? Will I feel like a freak? Will I feel distorted and unfeminine? Will I have "phantom breast," strange sensations and pains in a body part that no longer exists? What will others think? How much does a breast define a woman?*

When you have not yet experienced something, all these questions are unanswerable. I tried to remind myself that this was not an elective or cosmetic procedure. It was a necessary step on the road to survival. I had no choice, so all I could do was to face it head-on, with courage.

My friend Mary reminded me of the Amazons of mythology, the beautiful warrior women who cut off their right breast so that they could be faster and more precise archers. Perhaps I could take up left handed archery and put the loss of the breast to good use! She also told me of women who tattooed their chest to incorporate the scar into a beautiful design. I hadn't thought about that! What tattoo would I choose, if I got one? Perhaps the phoenix, another mythological creature, the fire bird that rises out of its own ashes.

Since the diagnosis, my life had crashed and lay in a smoldering pile. Could I rise out of those ashes and spread my wings once again. With the surgery still looming dark ahead of me, I did not know what waited on the other side, but for the moment, the phoenix seemed like a suitable symbol. I cried, though, and felt much fear, but also felt the peace of inevitability.

> *"I cried out in my affliction to the Lord,*
>   *my God,*
> *And He heard my voice;*
> *Out of the belly of hell, You heard the cry*
>   *of my voice.*
> *You cast me into the depths*
>   *of the heart of the sea,*
> *And rivers encompassed me."*
>
> Jonah 2:2-4

Rabbi Moishe

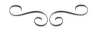

Rabbi Moishe was the next stop in my spiritual journey.

I was an adult when I came to discover my Jewish ancestry. An old bible given to me by my grandmother had a family tree of three generations of births and deaths, and my husband commented with surprise that "all the Simons and the Kuhn sure looked like a bunch of Jews," a hypothesis confirmed as fact when I next visited my grandmother in Romania.

As I drove to the other side of town to meet with the rabbi, I felt nervous. The reprobation from Rabbi Moishe could be double strong: not only was I not a believer, I was not a good Jew either. In fact I was barely even a Jew. Was the fact that someone, somewhere in the distant branches of the family tree, had been a Jew even count? Driving to meet him made me realize that I did not belong anywhere. I was not a Christian, not a Jew, not an anything; just a lost soul in search of a home.

Rabbi Moishe greeted me warmly. He ordered some tea for us, and after we sat down, I gave him a quick rundown of the events of my life in the past few months.

"I hear what you are saying," responded Rabbi Moishe when I stopped. "For a long time you have yearned for something spiritual and have wondered about it, but nine months ago you would not have wanted to sit here with me talking about God. What has happened in the intervening time? You have been struck by a terrible illness.

"The Bible talks about prophets. In biblical times, prophets were not fortune tellers or psychics who told the future. They were people who had a special relationship with God, who had the power to awaken others to the connection that they themselves could have with God and spirituality. Unfortunately, today we don't have prophets anymore. Today that role is filled by illness. It is illness that awakens in us a deep desire for something bigger than us, for a spiritual connection with the Almighty."

"But I feel that I am too old to have such a relationship," I responded. "I feel that at my age, you don't just wake up one morning and say, ok, today I am going to start a relationship with God. It's not something you think about, it's not an intellectual act. I imagine that faith is something so deeply emotional that it doesn't even lend itself to thinking."

"You know, though," said Rabbi Moishe enthusiastically, "that thoughts affect our emotions, so if we are open to thinking about God, that will affect our emotions and, with time, deep belief will evolve. For some people, there is an awakening, a sudden experience of some kind, but for most, it grows with daily nurturing and awareness.

"There are many paths to that spiritual goal; there isn't just one way to discover God. You have to start with an openness: You have to open your eyes and see what is happening right in front of you. The more open you are, the more you start seeing. God reveals himself through coincidences that have no logical or comprehensible explanation. Once you start talking to people, you hear amazing stories of experiences that defy all reason. God is present in those experiences. One day, when I was in Israel, I was talking to this man about coincidences, his name was Ya.., Cha..., I can't remember, I'll call him Simon."

"Oh, that's my mother's maiden name," I replied offhandedly.

"What?! That's amazing! You know why? Because I have never used the name Simon in talking about someone in my entire life. Why would I say exactly that name with you sitting here, and your mother's maiden name is Simon? Don't you think that's extraordinary? I think that's extraordinary! That's exactly what I am talking about! This is one of those coincidences through which God is showing himself!"

He proceeded to tell me about holy men whom he had known, who experienced coincidences on a daily basis. It was clear from his stories that being holy increased the likelihood of coincidences dramatically. His enthusiasm was infectious. I felt drawn into his circle of belief; I understood what he meant by strange coincidences, and, for that moment, I believed that there are things that happen that are outside our limited human experience.

"But what do I have to do to grow my faith?" I persisted. "Is keeping my eyes open and looking for coincidences enough? What if the coincidences in my life are few and far apart? What if I don't get any? After all, there is a world of difference between me and the holy men who have a relationship with God and who experience coincidences daily. Isn't there something I should be doing?"

"Yes, there is! You must practice being grateful. That is something we don't do enough of. When something bad happens to us, we focus all our emotional energy on one question: 'Why me?' We want to understand, and we are angry, and we want answers. We want someone to blame - God, the Universe - someone to hold responsible for our misfortune. But do we ask 'why me?' when things are going well, when our children are happy, when we are successful in business, when life seems to be charmed? Those things we attribute to our hard work and self-control and cleverness. We pat ourselves on the back and we take things for granted. We blame the Almighty for our hard times, but we don't give Him thanks for the good times. We take credit for those."

He went on, "We focus on the negative. A 100-point drop in the stock market fills us with anxiety and worry, but a 100-point increase barely registers emotionally. We are primed from birth to respond and react with intense emotions to anything negative. For the rest of our lives we have to fight that tendency and make an effort to move in the opposite direction, to notice the positive and give thanks for the good things that we receive.

"Take your situation. You have been very ill. To be pulled out to sea by a tidal wave of fear and doubt and negativity feels so natural! We all do that because it is how we are wired. But, even now, during this time of fear and darkness, can you think of things that you are grateful for?"

I didn't have to think long. Though I am often swept away by fear and confusion and doubt and anger and depression, the good things are there too: my family and my friends who surround me with so much love and compassion; my medical team whose attentive expertise is a powerful ally. I am grateful that I live now, rather than 100 years ago when a breast cancer diagnosis meant certain death; that I have the energy to work; that I have a job I love; that the sun is shining, the birds are singing, my cat is purring, my loyal dog is curled at my side, my cup of hot chocolate is hot and creamy. A million things, big and small, to be grateful for.

"Yes, I can think of a few things I am grateful for."

"This you must do every morning. Make your first thought be about the joyful things in your life because God is there in every one of them."

With that we parted, agreeing to meet again after I had thought about his words. When I got home, I went straight to the Bible. Was there something it could tell me about what I had learned from Rabbi Moishe?

> *"He reveals the deep and hidden things, and*
> *He knows what is in the darkness, and the*
> *light is with Him."*
>
> *Daniel 2:22*

For a short time, it seemed that a magic synchronicity existed between my feelings and every page and passage that I read. When I doubted, I found comforting reassurance. When I was glad, I found joyful affirmation. When I was sad and scared, I found strength and encouragement. But then it vanished as quickly as it had come. I painfully discovered that the path to faith was not a straight road nor were there short cuts and bypasses. I felt lost and confused and frustrated. The passages I read in the Bible no longer "resonated for me."

How does it feel to believe? Is it an all-encompassing feeling of peace and serenity? If I ever reach that point, will there be a quantum difference between the non-believing me and the believing me? Will I recognize it when it comes? The doubts and questions cycled through my consciousness with a tiresome inevitability. Often I had the feeling that this quest of mine was nothing but a fool's journey, a futile effort that would end in embarrassment. Short of a miracle, how can a life-long atheist, find God and faith? Those moments were terrible, the discouragement so heavy and so thick that it engulfed me in suffocating hopelessness.

> *"Cast not away therefore your confidence,*
> *which has great reward. For you have need*
> *of endurance, so that after you have done the*
> *will of God, you might receive the promise."*
>
> *Hebrews 10: 35-36*

I do not yet know how to pray. I meditate, I count my breaths, I try to concentrate and clear my mind. I sit quietly and calm my thoughts. But, then, nothing. I feel nothing. I wish I had a map to tell me that I am making progress. I think of Father John's words, that I do not need to struggle so, that all I need to do is be open and invite God in to lead the way. But, for me, talking to God is like talking to someone in another room, except no one is in the other room.

No one is listening.

I am just talking to myself.

I want to know that I am on the right path.

"What did you go out into the wilderness to see? A reed shaken by the wind?"

Matthew 11: 7

⁓

The day of surgery for the mastectomy arrived at long last. The surgery was a success. The remainder of the tumor was removed and with it my left breast. In its place, under the pectoralis muscle, a silicone expander bag was inserted, since I had elected to have reconstructive surgery. I had seen pictures of reconstructed breasts, and the likeness to a real breast seemed surprisingly good. With the scar diminished by time and a nipple tattooed by an expert, a breast lookalike appeared to be a reasonable solution.

My breast was cut off; I had been sliced and cut and punctured. The pain medicine gave me nausea, and the Valium, intended to reduce muscle spasms and anxiety, made me depressed and discouraged. The two drains that removed accumulated fluid where the breast had been made movement awkward and sleep uncomfortable. I couldn't drive and I couldn't work. I felt weak and pathetic, engulfed in a sea of sadness. The recovery was an ordeal. I felt that I had nothing left in me.

Millions of women before me had gone through it and millions more were going through it now. Was everyone struggling so? Were they much braver? When others talked about their experience of cancer, all I heard was self-composure and serenity. They talked about their faith and the immeasurable confidence it bestowed upon them. Compared to that, I was a mess, struggling in an empty universe. I wished fervently for a deity that stood with me and gave me comfort when I was afraid. But that wish floated out into a dark and silent void.

> *"Come to Me all you who labour and are heavy laden, and I will give you rest. Take My yoke upon you, and learn from Me; for I am gentle and lowly in heart, and you will find rest for your souls."*
>
> *Matthew 11: 28-29*

Service For Healing

"Angela has leukemia," my sister called to tell me with disbelief. Her childhood friend had just been diagnosed with cancer, and she found it hard to believe that yet another person she knows has cancer.

"How is she?" I asked, "how is she coping? She must be so scared. That's so terrible! I just can't believe it."

"Actually, it's amazing! I just talked to her, and she sounds so calm. She is so sure that everything will be ok. I would be totally freaking out. Heck, I am more freaked out than she is. She is very religious, you know, and she has this confidence that her faith will heal her."

I thought of Angela and I thought of Father Maximilian the priest at the Orthodox church in town, where Angela was a parishioner, and I knew that I wanted to talk with him about my spiritual struggle. I didn't know him, but I had been told that he was wise and cultured and warm and accepting, and I wanted to meet with him as soon as possible.

Angela had already offered to speak with him on my behalf, and I looked forward to that, but now she was the one who needed comfort and reassurance.

"I am doing ok," she responded when I telephoned to ask her how she was handling the terrible news. "I was really scared when I found out, but now I am better. I pray a lot and everyone at the church is praying for me, and I feel at peace. Everyone's strength is supporting me and making me strong, and God is hearing my prayers. I know I will be all right."

"I haven't forgotten about talking to Father Maximilian," she added, "but it just occurred to me that you might want to come with me to church on Friday night for a special healing service. Four priests will be giving the service and praying for healing. I think you should come. It will help you. You can bring something that they can bless for you, maybe a scarf or a hat."

The idea of the healing service appealed to me instantly, though, I didn't know what to expect, not from the service nor from myself. I had no frame of reference to prepare myself for such an event, except what I had seen in the movies: healing services where the preacher touches the ailing, and they fall to the ground in divine ecstasies, only to get up and walk off completely healed from whatever ailed them. Somehow, I didn't think that would occur, but the

Hollywood depiction was all that came to mind.

It was cold and dark by 6:30 that November evening, and rain was falling when I arrived at the church. I expected the parking lot to be filled with cars, people coming to be healed and comforted, but only a handful were scattered in the lot. I felt nervous and chilly as I dashed through the wet darkness, second-guessing my decision to come. After all, I didn't even know how to pray yet. God and I were not on speaking terms. But, before I could turn around to leave, someone opened the door and invited me in, commenting on the cold and ugly weather.

And in a moment, I was inside, embraced by the golden glow of candles and the rich scent of incense floating in the air. On the altar, beautiful icons of saints and angels with gold halos reflected the light of the candles filling the room with glitter and brilliance. The priests' vestments, opulently embroidered with gold thread, glinted with the slightest movement. The service had started. I found Angela in the front row and I sat quietly next to her. I was filled with anticipation, but with some anxiety as well.

As the priests were chanting the scripture and the prayers, I could see out of the corner of my eye that people were crossing themselves. Should I go along and make the sign of the cross, even though I did not believe? Was it rude to stand there and do nothing? It seemed inappropriate to interrupt Angela to ask her, since she appeared to be deep in prayer. Then it occurred to me that I was wasting time with doubts and questions. I heard Father John's voice, "you don't have to struggle so," and I realized that there was nothing I needed to do in that moment, but let go of my tension and allow myself to be absorbed by the spirit surrounding me. And as I did, waves of sadness washed over me. After months of crying, I was surprised that I had any tears left, but tears were streaming down my face as I was listening to the priests' chants. They spoke of pain and suffering and a soul that is filled with anguish and doubt and of hope for redemption and of God's readiness to forgive all sins and the resurrection of the penitents who allow God into their heart. I listened to the hypnotic chant and felt comforted by the sound of my native tongue. I kneeled; I touched the priest's vestments as he prayed over the sick and suffering; I kissed the scripture wrapped in gold; I let myself be swept away by the moment and wished fervently that something magical would happen to me and I would believe.

Angela took hold of my arm and dragged me to the front of the church where people were lining up to be blessed.

"You have to be blessed and anointed," she whispered to me.

"But I am not baptized," I responded. "I don't think I

am supposed to. I don't even know what I believe or what I'm doing."

"Don't worry about it. It'll be fine. Can't hurt. But I will ask the Father."

As I stood there in line, waiting nervously for my turn to be blessed and anointed, I knew that I had not yet found my way. I felt apart and I felt alone. And I also felt scared. To participate in a sacrament, without being part of the faith, seemed like a frightening sacrilege. Hollywood images once again came to mind. But this time, not of miraculous healing, but of brimstone and fire. I wished I was not waiting in line, but there was nothing I could do. To walk away seemed impossible in that moment, an unforgivable offense. So I stood there and slowly advanced towards the priest, who said a blessing of healing for each person, while making the sign of the cross and anointing him or her with oil on the forehead, cheeks, and wrists. Then my turn came, and Angela asked him softly if I could partake in the blessing, though I was not a Christian or baptized. He hesitated a moment, to respond to a situation that I am sure he never before faced, then he nodded and said the blessing, made the sign of the cross over me, touched me with the oil, and then it was over. I knew that the magic I had hoped for had not come to pass.

I thanked Angela for inviting me and headed out. Just as I was about to open the large door into the night, an elderly woman stopped me and said, "I had cancer seven years ago. I was stunned when I was diagnosed because I never thought it would happen to me. I was a good person and I led a good life, but there I was with cancer. We think we can control things, but the cancer made me realize that we have very little control. We have to put our life in the hands of God and pray and that's what I did. I prayed that God be by my side as I went through that terrible time. And he heard me and he was there with me every step. I am healthier now than I have ever been in my whole life. I am strong and I thank God for it all. God bless you and God be with you!" I wanted to talk to her, to ask her questions about her illness and about her faith, but she mumbled something about needing to find her husband, and she turned and walked away.

I stood there, not quite sure what had just happened. Yes, I had a scarf on, but the average person walking by would have no reason to think that I had been through cancer. I had no breast cancer pin or ribbon on. It seemed odd that a complete stranger walked up to me and expressed the very thoughts I have been struggling with. *That was weird,* I thought to myself as I walked out into the night.

I felt tired, but at peace. I knew that the emotional

release was important, that I was probably still grieving over what the cancer had taken from me and all that I had gone through. Other than that, I didn't know what to make of the night's events. I felt sure, though, that I was no closer to finding God.

It was many days later that I remembered Rabbi Moishe's words: "Pay attention to coincidences. When you notice them, God is present." The face of the elderly woman came back to me and I heard her voice: "We have to put our lives in the hands of God and pray, and that's what I did."

> *"Thou art my hiding place; thou shalt pre*
> *serve me from trouble; thou shalt compass*
> *me about with songs of deliverance."*
>
> *Psalm 32:7*

Pastor Smith

"Mom, I think you should try this Protestant church in my neighborhood," my son told me on the telephone one day. "I heard that everyone there is really open and welcoming and that the pastor is a young woman who is really nice and warm. Maybe it will help you to talk to someone who is not an old, white guy." I called the next morning and spoke directly to Pastor Smith, who agreed readily to meet with me.

Before my meetings with the priest and the rabbi I had felt nervous, concerned with what they might think. This time I felt no worry. In fact, I was looking forward to hearing what a woman's perspective might be and what advice she would have for me.

"I would like to know about God," I told Pastor Smith after explaining to her my background and my search. "What will help me know that God exists?"

"God is present in every relationship where you feel love," Pastor Smith answered. "God's language is the support of the people around us. He speaks through the love and caring of the congregation and the friends and neighbors who support us when we are scared and anxious or going through a hard time. We are surrounded by that love, and that love is God."

"But isn't that just people being nice?" I asked. "I am a caring and supportive person; I do things for others all the time, not because I believe that God commands me or expects me to. I do it because it is the good and loving thing to do."

"You do not need to believe in God in order for God to work through you," she replied. "Love, everything that is good, is a manifestation of God."

"I like the idea of a God who is love itself," I answered, "but I cannot comprehend how a good and loving God could allow the terrible things that have happened in this world, since the beginning of time, day in and day out. This is an insurmountable obstacle for me. I do not know how to reconcile a loving God with the terrible things that take place all around us." I was not trying to be argumentative or a contrarian, but this, perhaps more than anything else, felt to me like an irreconcilable problem.

"God has nothing to do with those things. He does not cause bad things to happen. A tsunami that destroys a village, a tornado that sweeps through a town, a disease that robs us of our health and peace of mind are not God's doing. These terrible things that happen are caused by forces of nature that have nothing to do with God. They are not God's will. We are scared and upset by those events; we feel devastated or lost when terrible things happen to us, but God does not cause them. God is the one who supports us when we are down and gives us hope when we are desolate. He is a force of good and love. God hears our pleas and gives us comfort. He understands when we are suffering and gives us the peace that helps us find our way. It is through this relationship with God that we experience the wonderful feeling of love and support, not only when we most need it, but on a daily basis."

Her passionate love for God filled the room, every corner, every nook. I saw it in her eyes. Her whole being exuded it. I felt the familiar yearning when faced with someone else's deep faith and wished that I could believe like her.

"But," I responded, "God seems like a concept that we made up in our heads to feel better, to keep us from feeling scared. I don't know what God is and what it means to have a relationship with Him."

She looked serenely at me and responded: "Suppose I tell you about my friend, about how loving and compassionate and supportive my friend is. You understand my description and you imagine the relationship I have with this friend, but that is not the same as you having the relationship with my friend. You know what I am talking about when I describe all the feelings of love and connection that I have. But it is only when you meet this friend and you have your own relationship that you truly experience that love and connection."

"But how do I come to a point where I have that kind of relationship? I want to believe, not intellectually, not in a mild or milquetoast kind of way. I wish I could believe fervently and passionately. I have started to read the Bible, and I always enjoy it, but it feels no different than anything else I might read that I enjoy. I do not experience any feelings of reverence. I read this or that story or chapter with interest, but that is all I experience, interest in a good story. I would like to read it and feel the magic of belief, but I fear that is beyond my reach at my age, at this point in my life."

"You don't have to be of any particular age to believe. Belief is open to all ages. In fact, there are plenty of cases in the Bible in which people started to believe as adults. Take Paul, for example. He was not a believer in Jesus and he persecuted the early Christians with great fervor. But the Bible tells us how one day he saw the resurrected Christ in a great light and he was struck blind by that vision. When his vision was restored three days later, he became a devout believer and a fervent Christian missionary who went on to found many churches."

"How do I know if faith grows in me? How does faith feel?"

"Different people have different feelings: calmness, confidence, hope, optimism. For me, when I feel closest to God and my feelings are most powerful, I feel a burning heart. There is this passage in the Bible where these people are in the presence of Christ, but do not realize who He is. When He leaves they find out that He was Christ, the Son of God, and they say 'Why didn't we realize that? We should have known from the burning heart we were feeling.' That is how I feel when I am in the presence of God. But as I say, it is a very individual feeling.

"I think that it would help if you prayed. Prayer is a personal conversation with God, a way for you to reach for him. But you must be gentle with yourself and allow it to grow without feeling frustrated with yourself. It might also help you to attend some services, perhaps try different churches, to see what you need, what feels right for you. I think that will give you some answers."

We sat silently a few moments, as her words settled and the conversation came to an end. Outside her window, birds were chirping noisily, and the afternoon sun was shining brightly.

"Is it ok if we pray?" she asked me gently. I agreed readily because, even though I did not know where I stood and what I believed, a personal prayer with someone who has a direct line of communication with God couldn't hurt. She held my hands as we bowed heads:

"Dear God, please bless this meeting and stand with us as we search and struggle with our pain. Give us guidance and help us feel Your love. We stand before You, with our hearts full of love, because You are love and You give us the support we need in our times of hardship. Please help Dana find the peace that she is searching for and help her feel Your loving presence so that she may know You and feel Your love. Please, dear God, bless Dana with health and bless her family and friends so that they may continue to give her the loving support she needs. Thank you, God, for all the bounty of love you bestow upon us. Amen."

My soul earnestly longs for Your salvation,
And I hope in Your word.
My eyes strained to look at Your teaching,
Saying, 'When will You comfort me?'"

Psalm 119: 81-83

Father Maximilian

I had waited eagerly for my meeting with Father Maximilian. Angela had described him as a deeply thoughtful and wise man, whose warmth and compassion had helped her deepen her faith immeasurably. I thought of him at the healing service and remembered his gentle face and the rich tones of his voice as he chanted the prayers and verses, and I was glad for the opportunity to speak with him.

"This has been a terrible year for me," I started, "a year of sickness and fear, cancer and surgeries. It has been very difficult, to put it mildly. It's true, I have had the love and support of my family and friends through it all, but much of the time I felt lost and alone. I felt a deep longing for something bigger, I yearned for something eternal, for the feeling of comfort that comes from knowing that we are not alone in the universe. But, unfortunately, since I do not believe in God, I have had no such comfort. So I come to you in the hope that you could help me, that you might have some advice for me about faith and belief."

"I am listening to you," responded Father Maximilian thoughtfully, "and you might be surprised that your words, 'I do not believe in God,' actually affirm the existence of God. Even if right now you do not believe, He is out there and He is in our hearts.

"We see God in the natural order of things. The manner in which things are organized and ordered in the universe reveals the existence of an intelligent being. Look up at the sky at night. Well, I guess these days you can't see the night stars so much anymore, but when I was young, I remember looking at the sky and would be breathless at the magnificence that was God's creation. Or think about the perfection that is a flower or the extraordinary way in which all the parts of a cell or an organism work together to make a working system. All that is God's design.

"There are those in science who argue that all these things are the result of millions of years of accidental mutations, of molecules colliding with each other. I don't see how colliding molecules can give rise to beings as extraordinary as we are. We have consciousness and an innate sense of what is right and what is wrong, and even when we choose to do wrong because we have free will, we know it. We have an awareness of good that is with us even when we stray farthest from it. It is not because of colliding molecules, but because we are the children of God. He has created us in His image. He has given us the ability to know right from wrong, good from evil, because He has made us in His image. God is eternal good, and we carry God in our hearts. When we stray from good, we feel it because we are apart from the goodness and love that is God."

"I guess I am really having trouble with the concept of God being love," I replied. "I have been reading the Bible regularly the last couple of months. I was told that reading the Bible and meditating on the passages I read would help me in my search. Well, a few days ago I was reading the story of Job, and what I read upset and angered me so much that I have not been able even to look at the Bible, let alone read it.

"I was familiar with the expression 'the patience of Job,'" I added, "but I never really knew the biblical story. I can't tell you how distraught I was to read that poor Job's suffering, the loss of his ten children, the loss of his servants and crops were all the result of a bet between God and Satan - a challenge by Satan, cavalierly accepted by God. I was so angry to read that God would participate in a bet in which Job, a blameless and devout man, in God's very own words, became a pawn in a game! God wanted to demonstrate to Satan that Job would still love Him no matter how many challenges and tests and devastating losses he faced! I could not imagine how a being that is eternal love could take part in such a bet. Would a loving parent do that to his child? I felt so much anger, even rage! I felt Job's pain, because in my illness and in my struggles of this past year, I have felt as blameless as Job, as much at the mercy of unknown and arbitrary forces as he must have felt. I am still distraught, and for the last few days, I have felt that my search for faith is a fool's errand which I ought to abandon."

"Yes, the story of Job is indeed a hard one to take, especially for the uninitiated, so to speak," responded Father Maximilian. "The Old Testament is not really a good place to start when you are trying to understand faith and God. The Old Testament is the part of the Bible that sets out the laws for what God expects of His people, and it can come across as stern and harsh. It is the early part, when man's relationship with God reflected more often man's fears than God's love. The story of Job in the end is really about resilience and faith and strength of belief that God does not abandon us and that the challenges, from wherever they may come, are more bearable when faith gives us strength."

I listened to his explanation, but it made no sense to me, and I felt angry because it seemed to me he was just making excuses.

But Father Maximilian continued: "Having faith and a belief in God does not mean that we are immune to sickness and disease. Our body is made of flesh, it has the limitations and weaknesses of all physical bodies. We are subject to the same laws that all creatures experience. In every one of us there is a weak link that predisposes us to certain illnesses under certain circumstances. Sadly, our body is weak, it is temporary, it dies. But what God gives us is the spiritual body of faith, the knowledge that through our belief and good works, we gain the eternal love and light. We find comfort in the knowledge that, though our frail bodies are but fragile vessels that easily break, our spirit is one with God and, thus, eternal. You have probably seen the studies that show that atheists have higher rates of depression, anxiety, alcoholism, and suicide than people of faith. To be an atheist is to stare, eyes wide open, into an universe that is empty and cold and unforgiving."

"When you say this," I responded, "it scares me because it reminds me of all the times when I have had that feeling. I've always called them 'my existential crisis moments,' brief peeks into that terrifying void, when I dared look and come face to face with the realization that everything I am doing is for naught, that it amounts to nothing beyond this brief existence we call life. I fear that there is no hope for me, that I am too old to move beyond my rational and intellectual concepts of God."

"I think the better place for you to start reading is the New Testament," responded Father Maximilian thoughtfully, "especially St. Paul's works. I think St. Paul's conversion would be something that will be meaningful for you. Here is a man who had no faith, who persecuted the Christians mercilessly, and then Jesus came to him in a great light and asked him "Why do you hurt me?" Paul was so overwhelmed by the great light that was God that he fell off his horse blinded. When his vision was restored, Paul became a devout believer, and he went on to do great works for God and for the Christians. His teaching about Jesus is deeply inspirational and will answer many of your questions. I think it will reassure you that it can happen, no matter your age.

"You are correct, however, that it is often harder to find faith as an adult than as a child, especially when you have had no background with faith or religion. It's like those water births. You've heard of them, right? Mothers give birth to their infant in water, and the infant is born with the ability to swim and hold its breath instinctively and never experiences fear. It is all smooth and natural. For those of us who only learn as adults, we have to overcome so many preconceived ideas, and fears, and handicaps. We stand in our own way too much, we think too much, and we are filled with fear and doubt when events do not match our expectations. We struggle too much, in short.

"I think you struggle too much. I see it in your intensity. You demand much of yourself and expect results in short order. And I imagine that you feel frustrated when results don't appear according to what you expect.

"You need to be gentle and allow things to unfold at their own pace. Imagine that your search for faith is like climbing a mountain. What you are attempting to do right now is march straight up and scale that mountain to get to the top. But that is really hard and fraught with hazards. You are likely to be overwhelmed by the challenge of climbing and lose sight of your goal. You end up feeling scared and uncertain and start to believe that what you are doing is pointless and not worth the trouble. I think you've probably had some moments like that already.

"What you need instead is calmly to follow the path that unfolds before you, circling the side of the mountain slowly and gently as you climb higher and higher with every step. And as you keep on, things that you could have never seen when you were at the bottom, will become clear and meaningful. So be gentle with yourself as you are going through this process."

But life-long habits are hard to break. No sooner did he stop talking, than I asked, "So what should I do? How do I climb this mountain slowly? What equipment, so to speak, do I need?"

"Well, as I said, reading the Bible will help answer some of your questions. Read the works of St. Paul. He will speak to you, I think, more than anything. I think praying will help you. I have a book of prayers for you that you can read in the morning for a few minutes and at night before you go to bed. Praying is our way of reaching for God and talking with him. God finds us when we pray."

"How hard can I possibly be to find?" I asked, half in jest, half in frustration, raising my arms and eyes heavenward. "I am here, God, I am ready to be found."

"God has found you," answered Father Maximilian laughing, "You may not know it yet or believe it, but He has found you. He is waiting for you to climb gently up that mountain. It might also help you to come to service, to be surrounded by the spirit of holiness and the spirit of God that permeates the Divine Liturgy. Well, I think you have a lot to think about, so we
could meet again in about 3 or 4 weeks, and we can
talk further."

The following Sunday I did, in fact, go to church. I arrived there promptly at the beginning of liturgy and was greeted by the smell of incense and the sound of singing. A handful of parishioners was sitting in the pews, already in prayer. The cantor was singing with a clear voice a beautiful hymn about suffering and penitence and forgiveness and eternal love. In the inner sanctum, the priests were praying and chanting. Father Maximilian was blessing the gold-encased Bible, and each priest crossed himself and kissed it. One of the priests moved about as he was swinging the incense holder, reciting blessings for the service and the congregation. Their vestments, though not the opulent ones that I had seen at the service for the blessing of the ill, were angelic in their simplicity: luminously white, embroidered with gold.

The service was long and arduous, with much standing and kneeling. The priests took turns chanting verses from the Bible, while the choir, seated in the balcony behind the congregation, sang lyrical responses and echoed the prayers. The chanting of the scripture, the prayers, the choir singing continued for over two hours, but at no point did I feel bored or restless. I felt
a calmness and serenity that I had not felt in a very long time.

> *"You shall sprinkle me with hyssop,*
> *and I will be cleansed;*
> *You shall wash me, and I will be made*
> *whiter than snow.*
> *You shall make me hear joy and gladness;*
> *My bones that were humbled*
> *shall greatly rejoice."*
>
> *Psalm 51: 8*

Rabbi Cassel

I drove to the opposite side of town to meet with Rabbi Cassel. My friend had described him as wonderfully warm and open-minded and felt sure that he could help me in my journey.

"He will be with you momentarily," his secretary informed me after ushering me into the waiting room. I looked around as I waited, only absent-mindedly taking in the surroundings: the framed art with Hebrew messages, the magazines about parenting, the pamphlets with information about Hebrew school. I was glad for a few moments to collect my thoughts. What questions did I have for Rabbi Cassel? I felt that I had grown since my first meeting with Father John. My early questions about how one prays and what one feels and what faith is all about felt childish and naive. I knew more now, but, in truth, I felt more confused than ever.

Every clergy person I had met with talked about God's eternal love and goodness. Yet, the story of Job still burned fresh in my mind. I felt Job's pain because I was Job.

I felt as blameless as Job, yet I had been stricken. The pain and suffering I had endured for months, the fear of cancer reoccurrence, though not on par with Job's loss of ten children and of all his worldly possessions, felt as arbitrary and unjustified as his agonies. The anger I had felt early on was once again coursing through my veins. *Why? Why did this happen to me? Why did I get cancer?*

"Hello, so nice to meet you," the Rabbi greeted me affably. "Forgive me for making you wait. Please come into my office." He already knew my story from my friend who had spoken to him of me, but I gave him a brief summary anyway, for no other reason than because I did not know where to start.

"You have been through a time of pain and suffering and hardship. That is very clear, but as you are telling me your story, I also hear that, through it all, God has been present. The neighbors who thought about you in your time of need and who brought you the food they cooked and visited with you were a manifestation of God's presence and love. Your family's love is God's love. He is the good we experience in our life, the support of others, the love they give us in our time of need."

"Yes, I agree. Through this ordeal, I have been surrounded by love and support," I replied. "But I always looked at it as kindness and charitableness: my friends and my family being there for me during a time of crisis, as I have been there for them during their times of need. How could it be God, when I do not even believe in God?"

"Well," he replied, "often people think of God as an old man sitting on a throne, a benevolent grandfather who is kind and warm. When we think of Him as this grandfather guy, it is hard to imagine how He might manifest Himself in people's actions. But such a concept only reflects our human limitations. God is greater than anything we could ever conceive. Imagine being in a dark room, and a sliver of light shines through beneath the door. That sliver of light is all that we can grasp of God, but God is so much more than that. He is the infinite light on the other side of the door. So, when you think of Him as a light that fills all eternity with brilliance, instead of an old man sitting on a throne, then you can start to see how He might be present, even when you are not aware of his presence."

"I have been told before that God is good and God is love, but I have trouble accepting this," I told him. "I read the story of Job, and God was not good then. I don't see the love of God when I think of what happened to the Jews. Six million were slaughtered by the Nazis. The Jews are supposed to be His chosen people, yet He did nothing to help them. Where was God when the Jews needed him? Or when children are killed in a school here or in Africa or in Chechnya?

The Bible says that God made man in his image. But Man is the Jew and Man is the Nazi as well. If God is all good, how is Man made in His image, when Man is a mixture of good and bad? I do not understand it and I cannot move past this roadblock."

"You are bringing up many things that have been argued over by clergy and philosophers for centuries. First, I want to tell you that the story of Job is not meant to be taken literally and it is not a story about God. It is a story about man and man's attempt to understand the challenges he faces, an attempt to make sense of events that feel incomprehensible. Think of the stories of the Old Testament as stories that teach us how to behave and act.

"As for the other points, there are many opinions that have been hotly debated. For example, Catholics believe that people are born in sin and that sin is part of them and that baptism washes away that sin. I think that people are born a clean slate, but they have tendencies for good and evil; what they nurture in their life will determine what kind of person they will become. Hitler was born a clean slate, but he nurtured the evil side of himself, so his actions reflected that evil.

"We do not know why God does not take a more active role on earth. People question his existence because he does not intervene to prevent tragic events from happening. I think God made the world, but after that he stepped back and let things unfold on their own— "You are free to move about the cabin", as they say on airplanes. He does not intervene or interfere. We are free to make our decisions and conduct our lives. Perhaps God is not omniscient. He does not know my thoughts, for example, which means that he does not know what I am about to do. That would explain why he does not intervene when we feel that an omniscient, loving God should. Keep in mind, though, that all suppositions about God, everything we think we know about God, is but a drop in the endless ocean of that which is God.

"I can tell you, too, that I know that God's support is in my life, that I could not do this work without that support. I am not strong enough to face life without God. Last year, I buried a child. I could not have done that and supported the family without God at my side. He is with me in all I do, and that gives me the comfort and knowledge that I can face whatever life brings.

"It might help you to join us for the Torah discussion group that we have every Thursday morning. You would see that you are not alone in your doubts. Even people who believe have doubts. Most people have periods when they question God or struggle to be with God in a way that is meaningful to them. There is even one man in the group who is not a believer, but he comes, faithfully, every week, because he wants answers. I don't know if he will ever find the answers that he is looking for, but he keeps coming."

"Where does that leave me?" I asked, a little panicked by the things he had said, "I don't know where I am going. I don't know how I will know when I will get there. I don't know what I am looking for or how I will know that I have found it, if I do find it. How long do I keep on? How will I know that I have reached the end?"

"I don't know either. I wish I could answer those questions for you, but I cannot. But I do think you owe it to yourself to continue on this journey that you have started. It is clearly very meaningful to you, and to stop would be a terrible mistake. I am quite certain that you will know when you have reached the end, but what you will find, that, I do not know."

With that, the time was up and I thanked him for his time and words. He extended an invitation again for me to come to the discussion group whenever I was in the neighborhood.

I was glad for the long drive home because I needed time to think about my conversation with Rabbi Cassel. He was the first clergy person that made me feel even more confused than I already was. He spoke of God's love and support, yet he seemed to be surprisingly doubtful. He thought that perhaps God was not omniscient, that he did not take an active role in the life of man. I felt closer to Rabbi Cassel than any of the other clergy with whom I had met. His lack of certainty felt reassuring because it was so familiar and it reflected so much my struggle, yet it was unsettling as well. What kind of God would it be who did not know and was not involved? In what way would such a God be helpful? I realized, then, that the God I was looking for was a personal God, so to speak, a God that took interest in my woes, a God that could offer the salvation and redemption and everlasting life that Father John and Father Maximilian and the priests at the orthodox church talked about, and that Pastor Smith held close to her heart. And with that clarity came utter hopelessness because I could imagine myself believing in a Buddhist God, one that is the river and the sky and the flowers of the field and the mountains and the stars. I could imagine such a God, but a personal God, who listens to prayers, and gives support, and has an interest in what happens to us, that I could not comprehend. And yet that was what I desperately yearned for.

> *"Trust in God with all your heart,*
> *And do not exalt your own wisdom.*
> *In all your ways know wisdom,*
> *That she may cut a straight path for you;*
> *And your foot will not stumble.*

Do not rely on your own discernment,
But fear God, and turn away from every evil.
Then there shall be healing for your body
And care for your bones."

Proverbs 3: 5-8

The Ghost in the Machine

With chemo behind me, I had a brief respite, a time without appointments, without doctors, without treatment. I had forgotten how "normal" felt! To go about one's day, to run errands, to work, to walk the dog, to do the countless things one does from morning till night felt thrillingly carefree. I had been told that it is scary to be done and be suddenly cut loose from the reassuring safety net of chemo and doctors' appointments. But for me, relief was what I mostly felt; and numbness. Nine months of surgery and treatment felt strangely unreal and eerie. Those early periods of anguish and despair felt distant and abstract. It was as though it had been someone else who had experienced them.

But the respite was short-lived. Before I could grow accustomed to this newfound freedom, preparations started for the next phase of my battle with cancer: radiation. The first appointment was a dry run, after precise measurements had been taken to ensure that the radiation was delivered in exact quantities, to the correct places, at the right angles to the chest and scar area. The first of thirty sessions was scheduled a week later, and just like that, I embarked on the next phase of this terrible journey, which, much to my surprise, felt more disturbing than anything else I had been through before.

"Good morning," said the technician who came into the waiting room to get me. "We are ready for you."

"I am so nervous," I confessed, as we walked to the radiation room, though in fact I felt far beyond nervous. I was terrified.

"Oh, there is nothing to be afraid of. You will see; you won't feel a thing," he added with a cheerful smile.

We stepped into the radiation room, white and stark and brightly lit. In the middle was a gurney-like bed of uncovered metal with straps and attachments to position the arm at specific angles, allowing the radiation to reach the lymph nodes in the armpit. At the head, a large machine with three outstretched arms hovered as though ready to engulf and liquefy anyone brave enough or foolish enough to lie within its reach. Ominous humming and whirring and buzzing noises emanated from the machine, making the prospect of lying in its grasp that much more unnerving.

I was directed to lie on the gurney, cold and hard against my back. On the ceiling above my head was a lit up scene of a Caribbean beach, with azure blue waters, white sands, clear skies, coconut trees blowing gently in the soft breeze, rustic cabanas where a tired vacationer might rest languidly in the shade. Another time I would have found the scene lovely and reminiscent of my trips to Mexico, but this time I felt it mocking me and taunting me. On this frigid February day, in a cold room, on a hard metal table, under glaring fluorescent lights, I could not have been farther from that scene! The technician strapped my feet together, and positioned my arm in the armrest above my head so I would not move. He pushed and pulled my body until I was in the exact position needed.

"Ok, we're ready," he announced as he left the room. The whirring of the machine increased in pitch and speed and the arms began to rotate slowly into position. I felt my heart speed up, in sync with the machine. One of the arms, with a large round disk and a glass window on the underside, passed above me and stopped in line with my underarm. I heard a rapid clicking sound and knew that the first radiation treatment had started. I felt cold and afraid and I wanted to cry as the whirring and clicking continued for what seemed like an eternity. I wished that I could see the waves of radiation. I was sure that it would help me to see them hitting my skin. As it was, I felt nothing and saw nothing, yet that nothingness was far more frightening than the bags of chemicals in the IV that had entered my body during chemo.

Then it stopped, and, once again, the arms rotated around me, with the disk stopping above my chest. This time I counted the buzzing sound, to keep myself anchored to something, though it was only to the fleeting time. "1, 2, 3, 4… 22, 23, 24, 25." Twenty five seconds, not the eternity that I had thought, but the knot of tears was still right there in my throat. I realized that I had to get a hold of myself. It simply would not do to fall apart in this way for the next twenty nine treatments. And, as the arms rotated to their next position, I started to pray the only prayer I had learned to the accompaniment of the ghostly sounds of the machine:

"Hail Mary, full of grace, the Lord be with thee. Blessed are thou among women and blessed is the fruit of thy womb, Jesus. Holy Mary, mother of God, pray for us sinners, now and at the hour of our death. Amen."

The prayer occupied my mind; it gave me a little distance from the cold steel table and the whirring machine. And then the clicking stopped; the technician came back in the room and told me that I was done for the day.

> *"And there will be healing for your flesh*
> *And care for your bones,*
> *That you may walk confidently in peace*
> *in all your ways,*

And your foot may not stumble.
For if you sit down, you will be without fear,
and if you lie down, your sleep will
be pleasant."

Proverbs 3: 25-27

Fear and Trembling

Meredith, my longtime friend was coming to town. She had been diagnosed with breast cancer two months before I was, so we had spent the past year talking to each other on the telephone, comparing treatment notes, reassuring each other, commiserating; in short, a support group of two during those many dark months. Now she was done, chemo and radiation behind her, and I was looking forward to seeing her.

"Could you bring the oncotype report with you, so I could see it?" she asked the night before our meeting. The oncotype cancer test analyzed the genetic expression of the tumor to determine its characteristics, the benefit of chemotherapy, and the risk for recurrence. On a whim, I decided to bring the original pathology report, as well, to review and compare notes on the cancer and the results of the mastectomy. I had not looked at either report for months and I was not prepared for the emotional tidal wave set off by seeing that information anew. The stark facts, the clinical findings, the lab results, so barren and emotionless, made my feelings that much more intense: "moderately-differentiated infiltrating ductal carcinoma," "stage IIB," "metastatic adenocarcinoma involving one lymph node", "invasive carcinoma involving the posterior superior margin," "4 centimeters," "rubbery and lobulated," "serially sectioned." Descriptions and measurements that went on for pages! Were they all describing me? I read anxiously, uncomprehendingly, and realized that coping with cancer was a work in progress, perhaps never to be completed. Feelings linger far after the point of diagnosis and long after treatment is completed. Like with grief, the feelings hit when you least expect it, when you are least prepared. And that night, and for days after, I was once again gripped by fear and depression.

In fact, what had I accomplished in these months of battling cancer? My body was bruised and damaged and so was my spirit. My search for God seemed as fruitless a quest as the search for the Holy Grail. I could not comprehend the most basic doctrines that the simplest Christian accepted as givens. Once again I found myself railing against God, the God in which I did not even believe.

"The whole head is in pain, and the whole heart in sadness. From the feet all the way to the head, there is no soundness in them, only wounds and bruises and festering sores."

Isaiah 1: 5-6

Father Maximilian— Reprise

I headed to my second meeting with Father Maximilian with a heavy spirit and a deep sense of discouragement. I had no questions for him, only complaints about God and resignation in the face of futility.

"I have come to the conclusion that I am not making any progress. No change has taken place in me. I have been going to church, I think I've been there every Sunday, in fact, and I have been reading the Bible and prayer book you gave me almost every day— probably I have been more devout than many a good Christian. But acting devout is not the same as being devout. I enjoy church a great deal and look forward to the service every Sunday. It is so beautiful: the singing, the chanting, the icons, the smell of the incense, it's all wonderful. But is that enough? I am not there to be entertained, yet that's how I feel. Every Sunday that I come, I think at the end, 'that was so lovely, I really enjoyed that. The singing was so beautiful!' But I might make the same comments at the end of a show or good musical that I enjoyed.

"I am coming to the conclusion that I am probably far too set in my ways to change. It's sad, but probably true. This is a fool's errand for me, and I must call an end to it. I am a person of science, trained to rely on observation and testing. Any hypothesis needs to be verified through careful gathering of evidence. To believe in God is to turn away from all that, to abandon the scientific method and take a leap of faith that God exists, that he created everything, that Jesus is the Son of God, that he is born of the Virgin Mary, that there is life after death and salvation through redemption. Even as I list all this for you, I realize how insurmountable an obstacle this is for me. Try as I might, my mind just cannot grasp these statements. I understand the words, of course, but I cannot comprehend."

Father Maximilian listened attentively, clearly troubled by my distress and vehement tone. "Indeed, you are speaking for generations of materialists who argue that the only thing that exists is matter in its various manifestations, and all phenomena, including consciousness, emotions, thoughts, and desires are all the result of interacting molecules and chemicals. Yet you just told me how you appreciate the Sunday Liturgy. You clearly have a keen sense of beauty because I agree with you: the liturgy is indeed beautiful. But is this appreciation the result of interacting molecules of sodium and calcium and potassium or whatever other chemicals? How could it be possible that molecules, in whatever proportion or complexity, could give rise to this thought that the liturgy is beautiful. Yet, that's what materialists would have us believe!

He went on, "Unfortunately, you grew up under communism, and communism was all about materialism. God was dead and materialism and the Party were everything. That was your experience! And add to that the fact that everyone in your family was an atheist, so there was no one to give you an alternative.

"You value reason and you want explanations that make sense to you. But think about this: we and the monkeys and the dogs and the mice are made up of the same chemicals and molecules. Yet we are the only ones who have a moral sense, an aesthetic sense, a charitable sense. Why? If the materialists are right, then a dog off the street should have the same feelings about the Sunday service that you do. But I think you will agree that it is not the case. We have consciousness because we were created in God's image. What makes us different from the other creatures is that we have a soul that puts us in a different category from them." With that, Father Maximilian sat back in his chair, waiting for a reply.

"Ok," I answered, "suppose I got to a point where I accepted that there is a Creator, a being that got the ball rolling, so to speak, with the universe. There is a whole lot of difference, though, between that and accepting that there was a man named Jesus Christ who was actually the Son of God, in fact he was God, and that he was born from a virgin, and then when he was 33, he was killed and was resurrected and ascended to Heaven. How could that be? That, I cannot understand. I know that Christ was a real person, but everything else doesn't make sense to me. It defies all reason."

"I see, you are also a spokesperson for rationalism. You believe that reason is the chief source of knowledge: if it defies reason, it cannot possibly be real. So between rationalism and materialism, you have painted yourself into a small corner. You know, though, that many key claims of materialism have to be taken on faith, such as how life started, or how the first microorganisms in the primordial soup evolved to become human. That takes some serious faith to believe. So faith is not just the purview of religion.

"But you were talking about Jesus and how you cannot believe that he is God incarnate. One time I was talking to a young man who was having trouble with the divinity of Christ, kind of like you. Well, that day there happened to be a spider in the corner of the room, and I pointed it out to him. 'See that spider? I would like you to ask it to come down here and spin a web closer to the window where all the irritating flies congregate. How would you do it?' 'Well,

of course I can't do it,' said my young friend, 'he's a spider. We can't communicate.' So I said, 'Precisely! Either you have to become a spider or it has to become a human, which is exactly what God's solution was. He sent His Son as an incarnation of Himself so that He may communicate with man.' God, in
His infinite love for man, His creation, wanted to give him a chance to redeem himself. Through temptation, man lost Paradise and, with that, eternal life. But God, in His eternal love, sent His Son who paid with his life
for man's fall, and by doing that, he earned man's redemption."

I could feel the frustration welling up inside me. "If I think of what you say as a fairy tale, then it's all good because it's a beautiful story. But if I think of it as reality, something that really happened, that just frustrates me because it is incomprehensible to me. I think that I have to come to terms with the fact that this thing I am doing is absurd and pointless. I have to accept that it is not possible for me to overcome my history. I really am like those kittens who had their eyes sewn shut early in their life and never could see, even after the stitches were removed."

"It occurs to me as I am listening to you," said Father Maximilian, "that you are a very stubborn person. You hold stubbornly to your belief that your past defines you. Our pasts define us only insofar as we continue to act on beliefs acquired in the past. Once we step outside those confines and open our hearts and minds to new beliefs, extraordinary things can happen.

"I also think you push yourself too hard. You need to relax and allow things to unfold at a gentler pace. Keep coming to church. Much good will come from that."

And then, he suggested that we pray together. We bowed our heads as we faced an icon of Mary and the baby Jesus, and Father Maximilian prayed:

"God, we give you thanks for this day. We confess to you our errors and our successes, our feelings and our doubts, our satisfactions and dissatisfactions. Give us the patience and courage to bear the burdens that confront us. Give us the faith to change our ways in this world so that we may serve you more faithfully.
Allow us to gain clarity in our thinking through the light you shine in our life through your eternal love. Help Dana find peace in this journey and help her see that you are present in this world and in her heart. Amen."

> *"Therefore if any man be in Christ, he is a new creation: old things are passed away; behold, all things are become new."*
>
> *2 Corinthians 5:17*

Nathan

A few days later I met with Nathan.

I had heard stories about Nathan from my son and my sister, who had known him in years past and worked for him while they were in college. They always spoke of him warmly, a man of kindness and good humor. Nathan had been a Buddhist for many years, but then he had a change of heart, and in recent years started to attend an Orthodox church and had converted. Nathan's story intrigued me. It seemed that he had struggled with something and that his story might have some answers for me. I was particularly interested to know how he reconciled his belief in God, who is supposedly goodness and love, with the fact that his wife had a terminal, degenerative disease.

We met for breakfast on a cold, sunny day. The hot tea was steaming in the cup that warmed my hands, as I told my story once again. I especially wanted him to understand how impossible it has been for me to grasp the concept of a personal God who not only created the universe, in all its extraordinary complexity, but also created man in His image, out of infinite love. I wanted to know, too, whether he thought there was any hope for me to find faith.

"I grew up Lutheran," he started. "I was very faithful, from a young age. The church that my family used to go to was right at the end of our backyard, so on summer days, when my friends and I were playing, sometimes I would just go into church— that was in the days when people left their doors unlocked and the church stayed open for the faithful all day— and I would just sit there and feel this sense of awe and wonderment. I wouldn't have been able to explain what I was feeling back then, but thinking about it now, I believe that was God's presence in the church and in my heart.

"Then I went to college and I was drawn to other religions. This was in the 70's, so a lot of college students were interested in Buddhism and the eastern religions. And I went that way too. There seemed to be such a free spirit and acceptance and openness about Buddhism; totally in synch with those times and that era. I was a Buddhist for more than twenty years. But then one day, about 5 years ago, Emily and I were sitting around on a Sunday morning, having coffee and reading the paper, when out of the blue I felt this overwhelming sense of spiritual emptiness. I felt this yearning for what I used to feel when I was a child, and I knew that I had to go back to church. I tried different churches for a while, then I found the Eastern Orthodox Church, and, right off the bat, I loved the beauty of the liturgy and the beautiful singing. And I loved the tradition. Did you know that the liturgy is the same as it was two thousand years ago— the same prayers, the same chants, the same ceremony?"

"I know exactly what you mean!" I responded, "The ceremony indeed is beautiful! I have gone to church almost every Sunday for the past two months and every time I go I feel this serenity and peace that I have never felt quite like that before. The couple of times I was not able to go, I felt a terrible, unsettled feeling of restlessness all week, as though I had missed something important. So the beauty, I understand! But, when you are talking about your faith and your connection with God, that is a struggle for me. It sounds lovely, I would like to have that feeling, but unfortunately it is not like a light that can be turned on at will. I often think of Paul or of St. Mary of Egypt. For them faith and conversion were sudden experiences. Not that I would want to go blind like Paul or live penitently in the wilderness for 40 years like Mary, but to have that sudden clarity, that vision, sounds wonderful! But, sadly, I think the circuits in this old brain of mine are irreversibly established."

"I can see the difficulty," responded Nathan pensively. "I grew up in a religious family, but my conversion didn't come easily. At first, I had trouble making myself go to church. Every Saturday evening I would think, 'ok, in the morning I am going to church,' but come morning the decision would evaporate completely. This went on for weeks. To this day I cannot understand what was going on with me. Then one day, I did go and I experienced again that feeling I used to get as a child, that awe and reverence—it was magnificent. Then I went regularly, and for two years I focused on learning everything I could about the Orthodox faith. I converted two years ago. Our church is truly wonderful! I have been surrounded by so much love and support, especially during the hard times of Emily's illness. God speaks his love to us and he speaks through us and through the people that help us."

Nathan's passion, as he talked about his faith and his love for God was riveting to me because it was so endlessly incomprehensible. Especially given his wife's illness! How could he talk about love when so much evil surrounds us, when he was facing the deterioration and early death of his beloved wife? And I asked him that, knowing that I was raising an issue about which he had likely thought a great deal.

"Man's fall from Paradise not only tainted him, but allowed evil to enter the world and with it, illness, suffering, decay, and death. Yes, the newborn infant is innocent because he has not had the occasion to interact with the world, but on a different level the sins of his father are part of his genes. You probably know about the Dutch famine studies with people who lived in the western part of Netherlands during the 1944 German occupation. Scientists are finding that children whose grandmothers lived through that famine are far more likely to have all kinds of health problems—heart disease, obesity, depression, even schizophrenia. So that innocent baby is not a blank slate, but carries in its DNA the history of the mother and of her mother before that and so on. Perhaps that is a way for you to think about sin. It isn't just what a particular person does, although that can be plenty sinful, but it goes back all the way to Adam and Eve, the original sinners that brought it into the world. Man didn't just fall out of Paradise, he fell into a state of sin.

"Sin is like the fungus that spoils a seemingly perfect apple. The apple is just an apple, but it exists in a world where death and decay rule. Think, then, what mortal danger man is in, who is so willful and filled with so much vanity and greed and so easily tempted. But God offers us love, redemption, and forgiveness for all our mistakes. He sent his son, Jesus Christ, to die for us so that our sins may be forgiven. Through him we can choose redemption, forgiveness, and eternal life."

"But," I persisted, "why doesn't God intervene when He sees all the suffering that we experience. Why does He sit by instead of helping? When bad things happen, could He not do something? It seems to me that for a being that created the universe, He has all kinds of powers at His disposal to reverse a terrible disease or stop a tragedy. I just don't understand why He does nothing! I have to say that this problem, perhaps more than anything else, makes it hard for me to take this leap of faith."

"I do understand your struggle. People have debated this, and atheists have used it as an objection to God's existence, from time immemorial. Why doesn't God make it nice and cushy for us? Why does God let bad things happen to us? How could He be the God of love if He allows terrible things to happen? 'Why me?' we ask. 'I am good, I don't deserve this.' We rail against Him when things are bad, but do we thank Him when they are good? Are we grateful?

"Maybe we should think of the bad things that happen as a trial. In fact, mystics and deeply devout people looked at the trials that came their way as opportunities to renew their devotion to God. Do you think we would grow much if everything always went our way? You are a child psychologist. I am sure you have seen children in your work who get everything they want and are protected from all challenges. You've seen what happens: they become emotionally stunted and self-centered and ungrateful. Trials make us stronger, and more generous, and more compassionate."

"I still don't understand though. How do you cope

with what's happening to Emily?"

"It's not easy, I'll grant you that! I have plenty of dark moments and sadness when I ask 'Why, God? Why Emily?' Just like you, when you were asking 'why me? why did I get cancer?' I do not understand. But then I think how often we do not understand our own motives, so how can we possibly understand those of God? So I think of Emily as a beautiful flower, a perfect rose that withers and will perish because of the sin that is part of the world. But I also know that though our bodies are of this world, and though we must all walk through the door that is death, on the other side our souls will continue on in eternal happiness."

"But I have been a person of science my entire adult life, and an atheist since the cradle. The things you are saying go against everything I have known with absolute certainty for as long as I remember."

Nathan's response came without hesitation. "Science and God are not incompatible! The scientific method is entirely compatible with a world that is created. In fact, science is possible because the world is governed by laws that are predictable and logical. Without that, all the carefully designed scientific studies would be meaningless. So, if you think about it, science by its very nature predicates the existence of God. It's just that the domain of science is the physical realm. Science can study the workings of the brain, the interactions of chemicals, the effects of various forces on bodies and matter, but it will never be able to explain how physical reactions can produce the mind. Our soul is not of this world, and science will never be able to understand or explain it. When you consider the extraordinary complexity of the universe, the perfect way in which it is fine-tuned to support life, it all clearly points to the existence of an intelligent designer. Can accident account for it? What kinds of accidental mutations could create the extraordinariness of life?"

I had to admit that I had no answer. My firm beliefs in evolution, in complete materialism, in a world of blind forces that, somehow, miraculously gave rise to life and made everything fit together perfectly had been shaken of late. But to go from that to accepting the existence of a supernatural being who lovingly and patiently waited for my salvation, that was a whole other matter.

He interrupted my thoughts with a few words of advice as we were parting. "Go to church. Keep going because that will help you, but don't do too much. You are pushing yourself too hard. I can see it in your frustration. Be patient with yourself! And pray. When you pray, you are opening your heart to God. Pray out loud, though, instead of just reading the words silently. That way you are not only seeing them, but you hear them as well."

"In this manner, therefore, pray:
Our Father who are in heaven,
Hallowed be your name.
Your kingdom come.
Your will be done
On earth, as it is in heaven.
Give us this day our daily bread
And forgive us our debts,
As we forgive our debtors.
And do not lead us into temptation.
But deliver us from evil.
For Yours is the kingdom and the power
      and the glory forever. Amen."

Matthew 6: 9-13

The Dream

I am sitting in the first pew...on the aisle, a few paces from the altar.... The church is filled with a golden glow and the haze of incense. I am aware that someone is sitting next to me. He is wearing a hooded cloak, and I cannot see his face. I feel calm and peaceful. It feels natural that the person is sitting there. He reaches his hand for mine, and I see that it is not really a hand, but something made of gold or light or brightness. I am not afraid as the light takes hold of my hand and I know that we are about to walk to the altar.

Looking back, that dream was a turning point, but even now I do not understand what it was. A divine sign telling me that it was time to turn the page? Or just my mind playing out by night what I struggled with so painfully by day? I turned it around and around in my mind throughout the day, a mental Rubik's cube. I saw the dream vividly in my mind's eye. I still see it now, as I write this. Dream analysis is a frequent staple of therapy, the highway to the unconscious, but clearly this dream did not need much analysis. But was there more to it than the average, garden-variety dream? In the end, I realized that there would be no answer. I would have to let it be, let it live within me and stop struggling, if only for one day. Whether it was a dream or a message, I would never know, but strangely, even allowing myself to contemplate the possibility that it may be a message, opened a door that revealed to me a whole new world of hope and light — an atheist at the divine threshold.

I was filled with a heady excitement all that day. For the first time I realized that, through all my discussions, with every single person with whom I had spoken, I never budged from my atheistic starting point. The premise throughout had been "there is no God," and everything they said was judged from that perspective and seen through that lens. Sure, I asked them my questions and I was genuinely interested in their answers, but, in truth, I never shifted my perspective or consider their position as possibly valid. I wanted to know what they thought and what they believed, the way an anthropologist might be interested in and fascinated by the beliefs of a newly discovered tribe, yet not for a moment did I give them credence or contemplate adopting those beliefs.

I realized then that if I were ever to come to a resolution, I would have to consider both options as possible. I had to regard theism on equal footing with atheism and I had to become knowledgeable enough to be able to make a decision that was not already predestined by my history. With that began a period of single-minded study, reading every book about God and faith that had been recommended to me.

I was most interested in books written by former atheists whose accounts of their conversion to Christianity were especially compelling to me. I read Warner Wallace's *Cold-Case Christianity* with great interest. He had been a lifelong atheist who converted and became a fervent defender of Christianity. He used his expertise as a cold-case detective to examine the evidence and witness testimony for the claims made in the Bible.

I Don't Have Enough Faith to Be an Atheist by Norm Geisler and Frank Turek, and *The Case for a Creator* by Lee Strobel fascinated me with their arguments for a created universe. As a die-hard evolutionist, I had never before considered the evidence for creation in such depth, and their claims were startling. At times I had trouble accepting their points, as a person who believed that the Earth is flat might, only to find out that it is in fact round. Their discussions of an intelligent designer gave me a new perspective, one that helped me keep "climbing the mountain."

I liked C.S. Lewis, who returned to Christianity in adulthood after having been an atheist since adolescence.

I read his *Mere Christianity* and then several others of his books. His eloquence and elegant writing style gracefully invited me into his world of Christian faith and helped me understand what it means to be a Christian.

Surprised by Christ by James Bernstein caught my attention because here was a man who grew up in a Jewish family and not only converted to Christianity, but became an Eastern Orthodox priest!

And when doubts returned, as they seemed inevitably to do, I turned to early Christian mystics who had the power to soothe with their passionate love for God. *The Cloud of Unknowing*, written by an unknown English country parson, and *Dark Night of the Soul* by St. John of the Cross reassured and comforted me when I was gripped by doubts. They had no need to prove the existence of God. They simply knew; their mystical knowledge of God guided them to the light. I let them guide me as well.

Every book I read made me thirst for more. And as I read, I realized that I no longer approached my quest with an attitude. I no longer required some indisputable evidence or blinding light or awe-inspiring vision. The burning bush that I had demanded facetiously so many times when I wanted a proof of God's existence was no longer a necessity. What I wished for now was an open heart and mind and a true desire to learn what belief and faith are.

> *"If any of you lacks wisdom, let him ask of God, who gives to all liberally, and without reproach; and it will be given to him. But let him ask in faith, with no doubting, for he who doubts is like a wave of the sea driven and tossed by the wind."*
>
> *James 1:5-6*

As I went along, reading the Bible and the many books I had accumulated, I began to feel more often peace and serenity. I still feared the recurrence of cancer, and the nagging post-radiation cough scared me with thoughts of lung cancer. But when dark thoughts came to mind, I prayed for strength and for courage and found that the fears no longer held me in their icy grip. As the weeks passed, I started to think of myself as a believer, a strange and new thought for someone who had been an atheist not long before. I continued to hope for unwavering faith and clarity, but all who had been my guides in this journey had told me that doubt is part of the human condition. "Help me God with my unbelief" became my frequent refrain.

Faith

I had survived a long year of trials and anguish and tears. I wanted some distance from all that I had experienced, a change to clear my mind and find my new center. So, when I had the opportunity to take a trip to Spain and visit family, I seized it without a moment's hesitation. I was sure that I would find the change of scenery refreshing, but what I found instead was faith.

Having grown up in Europe, I had experienced its rich history first hand. I had seen the churches and cathedrals and marveled at the architectural magnificence and the extraordinary skill of the builders. In those days, the achievement and artistry was all that I saw. I did not see the faith that had inspired them nor the love for God that motivated their dedication. But on this trip, in every town and around every corner, with "new" eyes, I discovered centuries-old churches with relics of saints that to this day inspire reverence and piety. Everywhere I went, churches large and small, all had reliquaries. Saintliness was not just a word or a concept, but a real presence that inspires and guides the people today as much as it did a thousand years ago. I felt the saintly presence all around me.

I felt reverence in the tiny Church of the Holy Cross in Najera, where peaceful silence reigned. I prayed there a long time, alone in the quiet dimness, where the only light filtered through the stained glass windows high above. I prayed in the small alcove where a larger-than-life statue of the crucified Jesus hanged, real hair partly covering His anguished face. I looked into His face, and touched His foot, and prayed for clarity and faith. And in that moment, something flickered, high above, across the window of the alcove. I saw it and, and in my heart felt that I had been heard.

I felt the holiness of Saint Emilian of Cogolla as I stood in the chilly chambers carved into the rocky mountainside where he had lived more than fifteen hundred years ago. He lived in that mountainside for forty years devoting himself to charitable works. His asceticism and holiness, his compassion for the poor, and the miracles he performed spread his fame far and wide. He wanted nothing for himself; everything he did, he did for God.

I felt the presence of Saint Dominic who dedicated himself, a thousand years ago, to improving the main road and bridges in La Rioja. He worked so pilgrims would have a smoother passage on their way to Santiago de Compostela, the final destination for countless pilgrims who wanted to revere the relics of St. James. That road became part of the *Camino de Santiago*, St. James Way. He cared for the pilgrims and performed miracles and served the weak and the poor. He lived a life of service to others and love for God.

I was surprised when I discovered that St. James Way passed right through the backyard of my sister-in-law's house. I could see pilgrims from my bedroom window as they walked by on their way to distant Santiago, and remembered how my friend Patty and I had talked about doing the walk together someday. Now, there I was, the Camino right in my own backyard. I felt it was a sign and was grateful for the opportunity to walk a part of it and follow in the steps of the countless pilgrims who had gone before me.

I started out with a determined step and focused mind, following the road through town, the scallop symbol of the pilgrim and yellow arrows as my guides. As the town grew distant behind me and the countryside spread out in front, my pace slowed and my focus shifted to the beauty all around me: rolling hills covered with vineyards; fields of bluish wheat sprinkled with poppies and chicory; small towns with church steeples rising gracefully toward heaven; dainty butterflies fluttering by; bees buzzing busily from flower to flower gathering nectar; murmuring brooks flowing over mossy rocks; croaking bullfrogs noisily greeting the day;

birds singing brightly in the sun. I took it all in, and my soul was full with all the beauty. There was nothing else I wanted. God had heard my prayer.

In the months after I returned home, I came to realize that I no longer stood at the foot of the mountain that for so long had felt insurmountable. And, to my astonishment, I realized that all along I had been climbing, and now breathtaking vistas spread out before my "spiritual" eyes. I saw fertile lands where faith and hope spring eternal and clear rivers that wash away the suffering and sadness. And as I looked on, I felt the joy of hope that there is more to life than meets the eye, that we are not alone, and that we are not the products of chance, living in an empty universe.

On good days, I see all this and I rejoice. But, though they are growing less frequent, bad days still snare me with traps of doubt, and I find myself slipping into old patterns of disbelief and frustration. On days like that, I remind myself that I am human—that doubt and disbelief are challenges that even the most pious person faces—and think about all that I learned. I think of all the books I read, of my battle with cancer, of my faith-revealing journey, and of all the company I had along the way. But, most of all, I remind myself that even on bad days, I am not alone because God is with me, and He will walk with me from this point on.

"The Lord is a shelter for the oppressed,
refuge in times of trouble.
Those who know Your name trust in You,
for You,
O Lord, do not abandon those who search
for You."

Psalm 9: 9-10

Notes

Bernstein, A. James. *Surprised by Christ: My Journey from Judaism to Orthodox Christianity.* Conciliar Press Ministries, 2008

Geisler, Norman and Turek, Frank. *I Don't Have Enough Faith To Be an Atheist.* Crossway, 2004.

Lewis, C.S. *Mere Christianity.* Harper Collins Publishers, 1952.

Lewis, C.S. *Screwtape Letters.* Time, Inc., 1961.

Lewis, C.S. *Surprised by Joy.* Harcourt, Brace and World, Inc, 1955.

St. John of the Cross. *Dark Night of the Soul.* Dover Publications, 2003

Strobel, Lee. *The Case for a Creator: A Journalist Investigates Scientific Evidence That Points Toward God.* Zondervan, 2004.

Turek, Frank. *Stealing From God: Why Atheists Need God to Make Their Case.* NavPress, 2014.

Unknown. *The Cloud of Unknowing.* Penguin Books., 1961.

Wallace, J. Warner. *Cold-Case Christianity: A Homicide Detective Investigates the Claims of the Gospels.* David C. Cook Publishers, 2013.

Personal Thoughts

Personal Thoughts

Personal Thoughts

PERSONAL THOUGHTS

PERSONAL THOUGHTS

Personal Thoughts

PERSONAL THOUGHTS

PERSONAL THOUGHTS

Personal Thoughts